CHAPTER ONE

Introduction to Migraine

Migraine is a debilitating condition that affects millions of people around the world. Those who suffer from migraines may experience chronic and intense pain, along with other unpleasant symptoms. In order to effectively treat and manage migraines, it is important to understand the basics of the condition.

What is a Migraine?

Migraines are a type of neurological disorder characterized by recurrent, severe headache attacks. They often cause throbbing in one part of the head, but some people may experience pain in both sides of their head. People who suffer from migraines may also experience a range of other symptoms, such as nausea, vomiting, loss of appetite, and difficulty concentrating. The exact cause of migraines is not known, but researchers believe it is caused by a combination of both physical and psychological factors. These factors can include food triggers, hormone fluctuations, metabolic changes, sleep disturbances, stress, and environmental or lifestyle factors.

Types of Migraines

Migraines are divided into two main categories: migraine with aura and migraine without aura. People who suffer from migraines with aura may experience strange neurological symptoms before or during an attack, such as distorted vision, flashing lights, tingling or numbness in the hands or feet, or speech difficulties. Migraine without aura is the more common form of the condition and does not usually involve these pre-attack symptoms.

People can also experience different types of migraines

depending on their symptoms and duration. Abdominal migraines, which involve nausea and abdominal pain, are common in small children and teenagers. Status migraines, which include continuous headaches that can last up to 72 hours, are rare but serious, and require immediate medical attention.

Symptoms of Migraines

Migraine symptoms can vary from person to person, but typically include throbbing pain on one side of the head, sensitivity to light and sound, nausea, and vomiting. People may also experience occasional temporary vision problems, such as blind spots and zigzag lines. Before a migraine begins, people often feel tense, experience mood changes, or develop food cravings.

Other common migraine symptoms include yawning, neck stiffness, irritability, confusion, and difficulty concentrating. Although migraines can be debilitating, they are usually not life-threatening. However, in some cases, people may experience more severe symptoms that require medical help.

Migraine is a condition that affects millions of people around the world, and understanding the basics of the condition is important for properly managing it.

CHAPTER TWO

Causes of Migraine

Triggers and Factors

Migraine is a common and debilitating neurological condition that impacts more than 10% of the population. It is characterized by a throbbing headache that can cause sensitivity to light and sound, nausea, and fatigue. Many migraine sufferers experience recurrent attacks and severe disability due to migraines. While the exact cause of migraine is still unknown, there are several triggers and factors that may contribute to the onset of a migraine.

Triggers are external and internal factors that can induce a migraine. Common external triggers are environmental stimuli, such as bright light, strong odors, certain foods, and even sleep deprivation. Other external triggers include stress, alcohol, or changes in the weather. Internal triggers are biological and include hormones, genetics, altered blood flow, inflammation, or a fluctuating body temperature.

The duration and severity of a migraine may be influenced by various lifestyle, dietary, and environmental factors. Poor sleep habits and stress are commonly associated with migraine onset, as is modern day artificial light. Other factors can trigger or aggravate a migraine, such as consumption of certain types of food or drink like coffee, cheese, or chocolate, alcohol, or environmental substances such as cigarette smoke.

An increasing amount of evidence suggests that nutrition may play a role in the development of migraines. Studies have shown that people who suffer from migraines may benefit from regular consumption of healthy fats, reducing intake of processed foods, and avoiding foods that contain tyramine or nitrate preservatives. Additionally, it has been found that limiting the consumption of caffeine and alcoholic beverages can help reduce migraine frequency and severity.

Humidity and temperatures may also contribute to the onset of a migraine. Some people find that they are more likely to experience a migraine during hot and humid weather, while others may be more prone to experiencing a migraine when the thermometer drops. Certain odious smells such as paint fumes or strong perfumes may quickly trigger a migraine for some.

Another important factor that can potentially trigger a migraine is an individual's hormone levels. Hormonal alterations can occur due to a change in diet or because of birth control, pregnancy, or menopause. When estrogen levels are declining, some women may experience an increased risk of migraine. Furthermore, a woman's migraine risk can increase when using certain types of birth control pills.

In addition, genetics can be a factor in a person's susceptibility to migraines. Migraines are known to run in families, and research suggests that between 30-40% of those who suffer from migraine have an affected first-degree relative.

By avoiding conditions and activities that may trigger a migraine, people may find relief from recurrent and debilitating headaches. Recognizing and understanding the potential triggers and factors of migraine is an essential part of successful migraine management.

Genetics

Studies have shown that several gene-associated pathways and mutations can contribute to the underlying biology of migraines. Variations in certain genes can influence the way a person's body produces and processes serotonin, a chemical neurotransmitter associated with migraine pathophysiology. Other genes implicated in migraine are those associated with ion channels and enzymes that regulate levels of inflammatory cytokines, modulating pain signals throughout the body.

A twin study conducted in 2018 revealed a 74% chance of migraine chance if both identical twins have the condition, and a 67% chance if non-identical twins have the condition. This suggests that genetics play a major role in migraine. The same study also highlights the influence of environmental factors, demonstrating that environmental components such as sleep disturbances, emotional stress, and lifestyle choices can also interact with genetic information to influence migraine predisposition and severity.

Further, research suggests that individuals with different forms of migraine may be genetically predisposed or associated with distinct gene clusters. For example, studies have indicated a gene associated with familial hemiplegic migraine, called CACNA1A, is associated with a high rate of familial transmission of hemiplegic migraine, a rare inherited form of migraine with visual auras, temporary paralysis, and other symptoms. Moreover, a rare gene mutation responsible for familial migraine with aura (FHM) has been identified in some families.

In addition to the genetic variety associated with migraine, certain gene combinations have been linked to prognosis and severity. For example, carriers of an APOE e4 allele (a variant of a gene for a protein found in the brain) have a greater risk of migraine affectation. Other studies have shown that people with particular gene variants that alter the serotonin and other neurotransmitter systems display higher rates of specific migraine types than the general population.

Genetics appears to play a major role in migraine causation and expression. While investigations regarding the complex interplay between genetic predisposition and environmental factors have shed light on how genetic mutations, gene-associated pathways, and other gene variants may contribute to the progression of migraine, further research is needed to better elucidate specific genetic contributions to migraine.

Changes in Brain Activity

Research in recent years has pointed to changes in brain activity as a likely mechanism for the cause of migraine. The first area of research concerns the brain's metabolism. When a person experiences a migraine, the brain's metabolism increases dramatically. This can be seen through regional cerebral blood flow (rCBF) measurements; the regions of the brain affected by migraine have higher rCBF readings than those of the brain areas that do not experience migraines. Additionally, brain scans have also revealed a hyperactivity in certain brain regions during migraines, including the thalamus and hypothalamus.

Further research has identified a link between cortical spreading depression (CSD), a wave of suppressed brain activity, and migraine headaches. CSD is characterized by a sudden decrease in neural activity, which can spread across the cortex in a wave-like pattern. During a migraine, the area of the brain affected by CSD is thought to cause the release of proinflammatory cytokines, which are responsible for the other symptoms associated with migraine.

Recent research has also suggested a possible role for the neurotransmitter serotonin in the cause of migraine. During a migraine episode, serotonin levels are reduced in the brain. This has been associated with increased sensitivity to pain, as well as decreased feelings of comfort and satisfaction. A further suggestion has been that neurons in the brain respond to serotonin by releasing substances that reduce pain, but that during migraines these neurons are not functioning correctly.

Stress and certain foods can affect brain activity and lead to migraines. Stress can cause an increase in the activity of certain brain regions, which is thought to be a precursor to a migraine episode. In terms of food, certain dietary triggers can cause a release of inflammatory substances which can lead to a migraine. Some of these triggers include chocolate, cheese, red wine, and processed meats. Therefore, it is important for people with migraines to keep track of what foods they eat, as this can help to reduce the number of migraines they experience.

CHAPTER THREE

Diagnosis of Migraine

Tests to Diagnose Migraine

As migraine is a complicated condition with many potential causes and triggers, diagnosing the disorder often requires various tests. These tests are excellent indicators for diagnosing migraine and assessing the severity of the condition.

Imaging tests are some of the most common ways of diagnosing migraine. X-rays, computerized tomography scans, and magnetic resonance imaging scans are used to reveal details about the structure and activity of the brain. These imaging tests can show any abnormalities, such as changes in brain tissue or blood flow, that may be causing the migraine.

Electroencephalography (EEG) is another way to diagnose migraine and other types of headache. During the EEG test, small electrodes are placed on the scalp and measure the brain's electrical activity. Abnormal electrical signals can be detected which can help confirm a diagnosis of migraine.

The patient's medical history is also taken into consideration when diagnosing migraine. The doctor will ask questions about the frequency and severity of the migraine episodes, as well as the patient's medical and family history. This information can be used to help detect any underlying conditions that may be causing the migraine.

In some cases, trigger identification testing can also be used to detect potential migraine triggers. During the trigger identification test, the patient is exposed to a variety of stimuli (such as light, sound, smells), in a controlled environment. The patient's responses are monitored, and any environmental factors that seem to trigger a migraine episode can be detected.

In addition to the above tests, laboratory tests can also be helpful for diagnosing migraine. These include tests of hormones, blood sugar, and other substances. These tests can be used to detect any abnormalities in blood or hormones that could be causing the migraine.

A Migraine Disability Assessment (MIDAS) questionnaire is also used to assess the severity of a migraine. This questionnaire helps the patient and doctor assess any changes in the patient's ability to function day-to-day. The MIDAS questionnaire is an effective way to monitor the progress of migraine treatment.

Differential Diagnosis

Though some migraineurs have an easily identifiable pain pattern and associated symptoms, this is not always the case. As a result, diagnosis of migraine can be complicated and often require a differential diagnosis to separate migraine from other types of headache disorders.

To diagnose migraine, the first step is for the clinician to take a comprehensive clinical history. This includes gathering demographic information, medical and psychiatric history, stressors, current medications, and severity and duration of the headache. A thorough physical examination should also be conducted to check for signs of infection or other neurological conditions.

The most important part of the diagnostic workup is to

exclude other conditions that may mimic migraine, which is known as the differential diagnosis. This includes conditions such as cluster headache, sinus headache, tension headache, and traumatic brain injury. Additionally, possible comorbidities such as depression, anxiety, and sleep disorders should be taken into consideration as they may be either the cause or effect of migraines.

A diagnostic tool known as the International Classification of Headache Disorders (ICHD-3) is used by healthcare professionals to assist in the differential diagnosis of migraines. This tool allows clinicians to make a diagnosis by comparing the symptoms to those that are outlined in the ICHD-3. The tool also suggests a number of specific criteria that must be met for the diagnosis of migraine to be made. Further testing, such as laboratory testing or imaging, may be performed to rule out other conditions that may be causing the headaches.

In addition to a physical examination and the use of the ICHD-3, clinicians may also order neuroimaging tests such as a CT scan or MRI to rule out any other structural abnormalities in the brain. These tests can help to identify any blood vessels that may be ruptured or narrowed, which can cause headaches. In some cases, a lumbar puncture may be done to check for the presence of bacterial or fungal infections. Spinal taps may also be used to measure the pressure in the spinal cord and for diagnostic purposes.

It is important to note that migraines can be difficult to diagnose due to their complex presentation and overlapping symptoms with other headache disorders. Differential diagnosis is essential to properly diagnose migraine and to ensure appropriate treatment plans are created. It is important to keep in mind that all clinical decisions should be made on an individual basis and should be based on the patient's symptoms, medical and psychiatric history, and current medications. Furthermore, diagnostic testing, such as neuroimaging or lumbar punctures, may be necessary in certain cases to help make a definitive diagnosis.

CHAPTER FOUR

Treatment of Migraine

Medications

Migraine is a debilitating condition caused by abnormal brain activity, characterised by severe head pain, nausea, visual disturbances, and sensitivity to light. Migraine episodes can last anywhere from a few hours to several days, and can be incredibly disruptive to a person's life.

There are many different treatments for migraine, depending on the type of headache a person is experiencing. In some cases, lifestyle adjustments and preventative medications may be enough to manage the condition, while in others, more aggressive treatments may be necessary. The most common medications used for migraine are triptans, beta blockers, and ergotamine derivatives.

Triptans are medications designed to abort migraine headaches, and are most effective when taken early in the attack. They work by constricting the blood vessels in the brain, thereby relieving the pressure from the headache. Commonly prescribed triptans include sumatriptan, rizatriptan, and zolmitriptan, but there are others available. All of these medications are taken orally, and side effects can include nausea, dizziness, and muscular aches.

Beta blockers are medications used to reduce the frequency of migraine attacks by blocking the stimulatory effects of the hormone adrenaline on the brain. Commonly prescribed beta blockers include propranolol, metoprolol, timolol, and atenolol. These medications are taken orally, and side effects may include fatigue, dizziness, and nausea.

Ergotamine derivatives are medications used to relieve migraine headaches, and are most effective when taken early in the attack. Like triptans, they work by constricting the blood vessels in the brain, thereby relieving the pressure from the headache. Examples include dihydroergotamine, methysergide, and ergoloid mesylates. These medications are taken orally, intravenously, or intramuscularly, and side effects can include nausea, vomiting, and drowsiness.

Other treatments for migraine include acetaminophen or non-steroidal anti-inflammatory medications such as aspirin, ibuprofen, or naproxen, as well as anti-nausea medications such as ondansetron and metoclopramide.

When selecting a medication to treat migraine symptoms, doctors will evaluate the patient's health history, risk factors, and pattern of migraine attacks in order to determine the most appropriate medication. It is important to remember that medications are only one part of a treatment plan, and that lifestyle adjustments and stress management techniques are important components of migraine treatment as well. With appropriate treatment, migraines can be effectively managed and the patient can return to enjoying life as usual.

Alternative Therapies

One alternative therapy option for people with migraine is acupuncture. Acupuncture involves the insertion of very thin needles into specific points on the body, known as acupoints. This therapy is thought to be advantageous because it can reduce the intensity of the pain, as well as decrease the frequency of migraine attacks. While the exact mechanism of how acupuncture works is not fully understood, it is believed that it alters the electrical and chemical signals that are sent to the brain, which can help to reduce headache pain.

Another alternative therapy option is aromatherapy. Aromatherapy is the use of essential oils, such as lavender, eucalyptus, peppermint, and rosemary, to help reduce the severity of migraine pain. The olfactory receptors in the nose detect the scents from the oils, which then sends signals to the brain to help reduce inflammation and help to improve mood. Additionally, the inhalation of the oils can release endorphins, which are natural pain-relieving chemicals.

A third option is biofeedback. Biofeedback is a type of psychotherapy whereby the patient is taught to become aware of their body's physiological responses to stress and pain. This can help them to learn how to control their physiological responses, which can then help to reduce the intensity and frequency of their migraine headaches.

Relaxation techniques, such as deep breathing, progressive muscle relaxation, guided visual imagery, and yoga, can help to reduce stress and tension, which can be beneficial for migraineurs. It is thought that by learning how to manage and reduce stress, migraineurs can reduce their risk for migraine attacks.

Massage therapy is thought to be effective in reducing the intensity of migraine pain because it increases circulation and releases endorphins. There is also evidence to suggest that massage can help to reduce muscle tension, which can help to reduce the frequency and severity of migraine headaches.

Chiropractic care can be beneficial because it can help to correct any misalignments in the spine, which may be contributing to the cause of migraine headaches. Additionally, chiropractic care often involves the application of heat and/or cold therapy, which are thought to be beneficial in reducing pain, as well as decreasing inflammation.

CHAPTER FIVE

Prevention of Migraine

Avoiding Triggers

Certain triggers have been identified that can trigger or worsen the condition in those who already experience migraines. It is important to recognize and avoid these triggers in order to reduce the likelihood of an attack and prevent further attacks in the future.

A trigger is defined as an outward environmental influence that can provoke or worsen a migraine. Common triggers include certain foods and drinks, environmental influences, stress, hormonal shifts, and certain medications. Identifying and avoiding these triggers can help reduce the number of migraines attacks experienced.

Foods and drinks can be an important trigger for migraine. Common food triggers include processed foods, aged cheeses, chocolate, citrus fruits, artificial sweeteners, foods with monosodium glutamate (MSG), and foods with tyramine. Many alcoholic beverages are also common triggers, especially red wine, champagne, beer, and whiskey. For this reason, limiting or avoiding these foods and drinks may help reduce migraine attacks.

Environmental influences can also play a role in migraines, such as bright lights, loud noises, or strong odors. It is important to be aware of these influences and to make sure to limit exposure to them as much as possible. Stress is also a common trigger, and it is important to practice stress management techniques, such as meditation, deep breathing, and relaxation exercises.

Hormonal shifts can also affect migraine symptoms.

During the menstrual cycle, some people tend to experience an increase in symptoms of migraine at certain times of the month. It is important to recognize these patterns, and if possible to make lifestyle or dietary modifications to improve symptoms.

Certain medications can also affect migraine symptoms. This includes certain blood pressure medications, oral contraceptives, hormones, and drugs that contain nitrate or ergotamine. It is important to talk to a doctor before taking any medications, as some of these can exacerbate migraine symptoms.

It is important to be aware of any long-term lifestyle changes that may cause or worsen migraine symptoms. This includes smoking or a lack of physical activity. Quitting smoking and increasing physical activity may be helpful in reducing the frequency of migraine attacks.

Stress Management

Stress can have a significant impact on the frequency and severity of migraine attacks. If stress can be managed, it can reduce the frequency of migraine episodes and decrease their severity. Stress management involves a variety of techniques such as mindfulness, cognitive behavioral therapy, exercise, and relaxation techniques.

Mindfulness is a practice that involves focusing on the present moment without judgment. Mindfulness can help people to pay more attention to their thoughts and feelings, and this can help them to respond to stressful situations in a more productive way. Mindfulness also encourages a person to consider the consequences of their reaction to stress before they act.

Cognitive behavioral therapy (CBT) is a type of psychotherapy that can help people to recognize their negative thought patterns and replace them with more positive ones. It also helps people to develop strategies to better manage life stressors. CBT involves developing coping strategies, such as reframing thoughts, problem-solving, positive self-talk, and relaxation techniques.

Exercise is a great way to reduce stress levels and improve physical health. Regular exercise releases endorphins, which are neurotransmitters that help to reduce pain levels and improve mood. Exercise can also reduce overall stress levels, especially if it's done consistently. Examples of exercise that can help to manage stress and prevent migraine attacks include walking, running, yoga, and swimming.

Relaxation techniques such as progressive muscle relaxation and deep breathing are known to lower stress levels. Adopting healthy sleep habits can also help reduce stress levels and lower the risk of migraines. Making sure to get at least seven hours of quality sleep each night can significantly reduce stress levels and the frequency of migraine attacks. People who suffer from insomnia should seek professional help for their condition.

In addition to these stress management techniques, engaging in healthy activities such as socializing with friends, listening to calming music, and getting enough rest can also help to prevent migraine attacks. Limiting caffeine intake, avoiding certain foods, and sticking to a regular meal schedule can also help to prevent migraine attacks.

Nutrition

The body of research pertaining to the impact of nutrition on migraines is growing, and there are a variety of dietary strategies that can be employed to reduce the symptoms and occurrences of migraine headaches. The first and perhaps most important step in preventing migraines is to identify and eliminate food triggers. Common food triggers include chocolate, aged cheeses, citrus fruits, processed or smoked meats, aspartame, MSG, and alcohol. Keeping a nutrition journal and tracking the foods eaten and the reactions experienced can help to identify any particular triggers. Additionally, avoiding fasting and keeping to a regular nutritional plan can be beneficial.

It is also important to maintain proper hydration and adequate electrolyte balance. Dehydration is a frequent cause of headaches and may trigger a migraine. Adequate hydration is key to maintaining good health, and it is recommended that individuals consume at least two liters of water per day. Additionally, ensuring adequate intake of electrolytes, such as potassium, magnesium, and sodium, is important, as these minerals play a key role in neurological functioning and maintaining balance.

Consuming a well-balanced diet is also crucial for the prevention of migraine headaches. Whole grains, healthy fats, fresh fruits and vegetables, and lean proteins offer the essential vitamins and minerals for optimal health. Consuming foods that are rich in Vitamin B2 (riboflavin) have been found to be especially helpful for reducing the intensity and frequency of migraine attacks. Furthermore, it is beneficial to reduce the intake of simple sugars, particularly those contained in processed foods and soft drinks. Refined sugars can lead to drops in blood sugar levels, which can also trigger migraines.

Incorporating dietary supplements into a healthy lifestyle can be beneficial for migraine prevention. Omega-3 fatty acids, magnesium, Vitamin B6, and Vitamin D have all been found to have a positive effect on migraine prevention. Magnesium, in particular, appears to be especially helpful as it helps to relax the blood vessels and nervous system. Talk to your healthcare provider before taking any supplements to ensure safety.

Finally, staying away from stimulants such as caffeine, nicotine, and other substances can help to reduce the frequency and intensity of migraine attacks. Caffeine can be particularly tricky as it can both trigger and relieve headaches. Thus, it is important to keep track of your caffeine intake and experiment to find your individual tolerance level.

CHAPTER SIX

Coping with Migraine

Managing Symptoms

People with migraine must face their symptoms on a regular basis, and it is important to learn coping skills to help lessen the pain and manage the side effects.

Pain Management

Pain is the primary symptom of migraine, and it can range from mild to excruciating. To reduce pain associated with migraine, experts recommend employing a combination of home remedies and lifestyle changes. Over-the-counter medications, such as ibuprofen or acetaminophen, are often used as a first line of defense against milder headaches. For more significant pain, prescription pain relief medications may be prescribed.

It is also important for people with migraine to practice stress reduction and relaxation techniques. Stress can be a trigger for migraine, and relaxing activities such as yoga, meditation, and deep breathing can help reduce stress levels. People with migraine should also practice good sleep hygiene, as lack of sleep or changes in one's regular sleep pattern can trigger or worsen migraine symptoms.

Other remedies to help relieve migraine pain include applying cold compresses or heat packs to the head or neck, taking a warm bath or shower, consuming caffeine-free beverages such as herbal teas, or drinking a lot of water. Additionally, it is important to find and avoid triggers that may exacerbate migraine pain.

Nausea

Nausea is a common migraine symptom that is caused by intense pain, motion, or stress. Treatments for nausea associated with migraine include taking anti-emetic medications such as promethazine. Eating smaller meals throughout the day and avoiding spicy, greasy, and processed foods may also help reduce nausea. Additionally, it is important to ensure adequate fluids are consumed to avoid dehydration.

Light and Sound Sensitivity

Light and sound sensitivity are common symptoms associated with migraine and may occur prior to or during a migraine. These symptoms can be managed with adequate precautions, including staying in dark and quiet rooms during an attack. Additionally, wearing sunglasses subtly tinted to block light and noise-canceling headphones can be helpful in reducing light and sound sensitivity.

Fatigue

Fatigue is another common symptom of migraine. People with migraine are more likely to experience fatigue due to lack of sleep or inadequate amounts of sleep, as well as the stress associated with the condition. To lessen the impact of fatigue, experts recommend getting adequate sleep, staying physically active, and eating a balanced diet.

Migraine is a condition that can be debilitating and difficult to cope with. It is important for people with migraine to be aware of the different types of treatments and coping strategies that are available to manage migraine symptoms. With the proper care and management, people with migraine can often reduce the frequency and severity of their symptoms.

Emotional Support

When faced with a migraine, it is important to remember that the pain and associated symptoms are real, and they have an effect on your mental and emotional state. Coping with migraine involves acknowledging and addressing the emotions that arise due to the disorder.

The first step to emotional support for those dealing with a migraine is to acknowledge that the pain and its effects, both physical and emotional, are real. It is important to create a safe, supportive space in which to express and process the emotions that come with dealing with a migraine. Creating this space can be as simple as allowing some alone time or expressing oneself to a trusted ally, such as a family member or friend.

It may also be helpful to find activities that provide emotional comfort and distraction. Simply engaging in a calming activity, such as listening to music, engaging in a favorite activity, or talking with a friend, can help to regulate emotions and mitigate some of the pain associated with the migraine.

It is also important to practice effective self-care. Emotional support involves taking care of the physical body, as well as the emotional and mental states. A balanced diet, regular and sufficient sleep, and regular exercise are all essential components of emotional health. Additionally, engaging in activities that reduce stress, such as yoga or meditation, can be beneficial for managing migraine symptoms and for improving overall emotional health.

In cases of chronic migraines or other forms of chronic pain, it may be helpful to seek professional emotional support, such as counseling, cognitive behavioral therapy (CBT), mindfulness-based programs, or support groups. Professional emotional support can provide guidance and strategies for managing and coping with the pain, as well as with its emotional effects.

Finally, it is important to practice positive self-talk and to focus on the positive. Reminding oneself of the strength and resilience of the body, as well as what one can control, can be beneficial when dealing with a migraine. Additionally, engaging in positive self-talk, such as praising oneself for being able to cope with the pain, can help to bolster a sense of self-efficacy and can make dealing with the pain more manageable.

CHAPTER SEVEN

Lifestyle Changes for Migraine

Dietary Modifications

Making lifestyle modifications is a key strategy to manage migraine. Dietary modifications, in particular, can play a major role in reducing migraine severity and frequency.

Dietary modifications involve making changes in regularly consumed foods, such as consuming fewer processed foods, avoiding certain food triggers, and increasing the consumption of certain nutritious meals. A migraine diet is typically divided into two parts: Elimination and Reintroduction.

The Elimination part of the migraine diet seeks to identify which foods might be causing or triggering migraines and then avoiding them. Common food triggers, such as processed foods, MSG, cured meats, aged cheeses, and caffeine are commonly identified during this phase. Additionally, foods that contain additives, such as preservatives, artificial flavorings, or coloring agents can also provoke a migraine attack and should be avoided.

Once the food triggers have been identified during the Elimination phase, the Reintroduction phase is used to reintroduce these foods back into the diet while assessing for a reaction. During this phase, only one food should be added back into the diet at a time in order to properly assess the reaction that may occur. If a reaction occurs, then the food should be completely avoided and other food substitutions should be made as a replacement.

In addition to avoiding food triggers, consuming more nutritious meals can also help reduce the severity of migraines. A balanced diet that includes foods from all food groups should be followed. This diet should include plenty of fruits and vegetables, lean proteins, and whole grains, as well as low-fat dairy products and healthy fats such as olive oil. Eating three balanced meals per day and avoiding large gaps between meals can also help reduce migraine severity.

Hydration is essential for overall health and is an especially important lifestyle modification for migraine. Ensuring proper hydration by drinking plenty of water throughout the day can help reduce migraine frequency and intensity.

Exercise

Recent research has demonstrated that regular exercise can reduce the risk of migraine and also reduce the severity and duration of migraine attacks. Specifically, aerobic exercise has been shown to improve migraine symptoms, such as frequency, intensity, and duration of migraine episodes. Exercise has also been found to be effective in reducing the use of migraine medications. Additionally, exercise may also help to improve sleep quality and reduce stress, two additional factors that may contribute to migraine symptoms.

In order to maximize the potential benefits of exercise for migraine, it is important to understand how to get started and create an exercise plan that is customized to your specific migraine symptoms. First, it is important to consult a physician before beginning any new exercise regimen. A physician can help to determine which type and intensity of exercise is most appropriate based on your individual needs.

Choose an exercise program that is enjoyable and that

you will be able to stick with in the long-term. Regular aerobic activity is recommended, such as walking, jogging, swimming, or biking. Additionally, it is important to include strength training, flexibility training, and balance training to your exercise routine.

Start slowly when beginning an exercise program. If you are new to exercise, it should start with low to moderate intensity. Then, the intensity can be increased slowly over time, with a focus on improving overall fitness and endurance over time.

It is important to plan for sufficient rest and recovery days when participating in exercise. Regular rest days are important to allow the body to rest and recover, which can reduce the risk of overtraining and injury. It is also important to listen to your body and take breaks when necessary.

Finally, make sure that you are finding activities that are fun. This will help to ensure that you stay motivated and continue to follow the exercise program in the long-term.

Sleep

Proper sleep can be a powerful remedy for migraine. Studies have found that even losing or gaining an hour of sleep could affect the amount of migraines experienced over the span of a month. Thus, the quality and quantity of sleep is important in preventing and treating migraines. Keeping a consistent sleep schedule, meaning going to bed and waking up at the same time every day, is a key factor in preventing migraines.

Proper sleep hygiene is also important to help reduce the

risk of migraines. A sleep hygiene goal is to protect the sleep environment, which can be achieved by creating a bedtime routine and a comfortable sleeping environment. A few tips to create a comfortable sleep environment include: keeping the bedroom dark, avoiding screen time one hour before bedtime, keeping the bedroom temperature comfortable, reducing noise levels, and minimizing distractions. Practicing relaxation techniques such as yoga, massage, or taking a warm bath before bedtime can also help one to fall asleep faster and have a more restful sleep.

Additionally, avoiding certain foods and drinks prior to sleep can help prevent migraines. Caffeine, alcohol, and certain food additives can make it difficult to fall asleep. It is also important to make sure that meals taken in the evening are light and not too heavy.

Exercise can be a great way to ease symptoms of migraine and improve sleep. Light aerobic exercise such as cycling, swimming, jogging, walking, and yoga can help reduce stress and improve sleep quality. It is important to note that exercising close to bedtime should be avoided, as late-night exercising can disrupt the body's internal clock.

Migraineurs should also start good sleep habits early on by avoiding napping during the day. Although taking a quick nap can be a good way to refresh, daytime napping can lead to insomnia and interfere with nightly sleep habits. If a nap is taken, a short 10-20 minute nap during the day can help improve alertness and energy levels.

CHAPTER EIGHT

Complications of Migraine

Migraine-Associated Vertigo

A more severe form of migraine is Migraine-Associated Vertigo (MAV), which occurs when a person experiences vertigo and dizziness along with the other symptoms of migraine.

MAV occurs most commonly in women with migraine and is thought to involve disruptions in the balance system of the inner ear. The exact cause of MAV is unknown, but it is believed to be the result of an alteration in the neural pathways between the inner ear and the brain. According to some experts, this alteration can lead to a disruption in the autonomic nervous system, causing vertigo and lightheadedness.

Some symptoms of MAV include a spinning sensation, lightheadedness, nausea, and a feeling of unsteadiness or disorientation. Other symptoms may include difficulty walking, blurred vision, confusion, and difficulty concentrating. MAV can significantly impair a person's quality of life and is often accompanied by extreme fatigue, depression, and emotional distress.

It is important to diagnose and treat MAV properly in order to avoid further complications. Diagnosis is usually done by a doctor performing a physical exam and neurological tests, such as eye movement and coordination, to rule out other conditions. Treatment options for MAV include lifestyle changes, such as reducing stress and avoiding triggers; medications such as antihistamines, antiepileptic drugs, or non-steroidal anti-inflammatory medications; and physical therapies such as vestibular rehabilitation and balance retraining exercises.

In some cases, an individual may have to take medications specifically designed to treat MAV. These medications can vary from anticholinergics and anti-inflammatory drugs to medications specifically targeting the vertigo episodes. If medications do not help reduce the symptoms, certain devices such as options for light and sound therapy, or virtual reality goggles, may be recommended. It may also be helpful to try certain relaxation and meditation techniques to help reduce the intensity of MAV.

It is important to remember that MAV is a complex condition and although treatments are available, the results may not be immediate. In some cases, the condition may persist for months or even years. It is important to work with a physician or healthcare professional who is knowledgeable in the treatment of MAV in order to get the most benefit from treatment. With proper treatment, people with MAV can manage their condition and lead fulfilling and productive lives.

Chronic Headaches

Another possible complication of migraine is chronic daily headache. This is the persistent pain and disability caused by frequent headaches. People with this condition are at a higher risk for developing depression, anxiety, and alcohol and substance abuse. This can lead to further severe complications, including poor work performance and social isolation.

Chronic migraine can also lead to medication overuse headaches. This is when a person becomes dependent on pain medications to manage their pain and ends up using them too often. As a result, the person experiences more frequent and more severe headaches and remains in a cycle of pain relief and pain recurrence. These headaches can last anywhere from a few days to many months and can be debilitating.

Migraine complications can cause permanent damage to the brain, leading to depression, anxiety, and other mental health problems. People who suffer from chronic migraine are more likely to experience cognitive deficits such as impaired memory and concentration. Chronic migraine can also increase the risk of stroke, as it can cause vasospasm. This is the constriction of the blood vessels, which can reduce blood flow to the brain and cause a stroke.

In some cases, surgery may be an option for people with chronic migraine. Procedures such as occipital nerve stimulation, nerve blocks, and nerve decompression can be beneficial in managing migraine symptoms. Surgery is not a guaranteed remedy for chronic migraine, and each individual should discuss the potential risks with their doctor.

Secondary Headache Disorders

A secondary headache disorder is one that is caused by or associated with a primary disorder. In this case, the primary disorder is migraine, but these head pain disorders can also be caused by other conditions such as head trauma or brain tumors. Secondary headache disorders are divided into two broad categories: primary headache-induced secondary headaches and secondary headaches brought on by other disorders.

The most common type of secondary headache disorder related to migraine is a chronic daily headache (CDH). This type of headache is considered a complicating factor in most cases of migraine and is diagnosed when a person experiences at least 15 headaches per month. Chronic daily headaches have several distinct characteristics, including headache intensity, frequency, and duration. Other common symptoms of CDH include sensitivity to noise and light, fatigue, depression, nausea, and dizziness. Treatment of CDH can be difficult and involves the use of a variety of medications, such as triptans, non-steroidal anti-inflammatory drugs, and opiates.

Another common secondary headache disorder related to migraine is tension-type headache (TTH). This type of headache is characterized by a band-like squeezing sensation around the head and is often accompanied by tightness in the neck and shoulders, as well as fatigue. Tension-type headaches are usually episodic and generally respond well to over-the-counter medications or lifestyle modifications to reduce stress.

A rare but serious secondary headache disorder linked to migraine is primary punctional headache (PPH). PPH is characterized by severe, recurrent headaches that are often associated with traumatic brain injury (TBI). The headaches are usually felt on one side of the head and are not triggered by physical activity, exertion, or other known triggers. The intensity and frequency of PPH can vary widely, and treatment typically involves a combination of analgesics and anticonvulsants.

Finally, there is a category of secondary headache disorders that is associated with various systemic diseases, including systemic lupus erythematosus, HIV-AIDS, and multiple sclerosis. To be classified as a secondary headache disorder, the headaches must meet the criteria of the International Classifications of Headache Disorders (ICHD) which requires that they be severe, disabling, and recurrent. These types of headaches are often difficult to treat and may require medications to manage the underlying condition, as well as medications that target the headache.

Secondary headache disorders can cause significant morbidity and disability and can greatly impact a person's quality of life. As such, it is important to thoroughly evaluate each case in order to determine the best treatment plan. Treatment of secondary headache disorders should be tailored to the individual and may include medications, lifestyle modifications, and psychotherapy. Additionally, it is important to be aware of any potential side effects or complications associated with medications used to treat secondary headache disorder. With proper diagnosis and treatment, most people are able to manage their secondary headache disorder and live better quality lives.

CHAPTER NINE

Managing Migraine in the Workplace

Talking to Employers

For those who suffer from migraines, it can often be difficult to manage the symptoms in the workplace.

In order to effectively manage migraine in the workplace, it is important to communicate with employers. It is important to let employers know that migraine is a real disorder that can have a serious impact on a person's ability to work. Informing employers about the signs and symptoms of migraine may help to ensure that employers take the disorder seriously. Additionally, it is important to provide employers with information on the treatments and preventative measures that can be used to reduce the frequency and intensity of migraine attacks. These measures may include changes in work environments, such as reducing light and sound levels, providing ergonomic furniture, and avoiding certain activities that may trigger or aggravate migraines.

Employers can also be educated about the importance of providing a supportive work environment. This may include providing flexible hours, allowing for frequent breaks, and avoiding stressful tasks that can trigger migraines. Additionally, employers may be willing to provide accommodations such as telecommuting or taking leave from work in order to manage migraine attacks. It is important to keep employers informed of any changes in migraine symptoms or treatments and to provide progress reports of any measures taken.

It is also important for those with migraine to discuss any workplace modifications or accommodations that may make it easier to manage their symptoms. For example, those with light sensitivity may need to limit the amount of time spent under fluorescent lighting or wear sunglasses in an office setting. Additionally, those with sound sensitivity may need to request that their area of work be relatively free of noise. It is important to be open and honest with employers regarding the types of modifications or accommodations that are necessary to manage migraine.

Finally, it is important to keep in mind that employers can be understanding of the needs of migraineurs and can be willing to work with them in order to create a productive and supportive work environment. It is important to remember that migraine is a valid and treatable condition and to take the necessary steps to communicate with employers and manage migraine in the workplace. By openly discussing migraine with employers and advocating for workplace modifications or accommodations, migraineurs can ensure that their needs are met and that they can continue to be productive and successful in their careers.

Work Accommodations

As migraine can cause intense physical and psychological distress, the impact of the disorder in the workplace should not be underestimated. Individuals with migraine are likely to be absent from work more frequently than those without and may have difficulty concentrating when at work. Employers must understand the disability and develop workplace policies to accommodate and assist employees with migraine.

The first step is for the employer to become familiar

with the illness. People with migraine are protected under the Americans with Disabilities Act (ADA). Under the ADA, accommodations should be made to minimize the negative impact of migraine and to enable individuals with migraine to continue to perform their job duties. Training programs should be established to inform supervisors and employees about the disorder, how to recognize its effect and help individuals with migraine.

Accommodations may include flexible scheduling, such as permitting employees with migraine to arrive late or leave early when necessary, so that they can get the proper rest needed to manage their migraine. Telecommuting or job sharing could also be options to allow individuals to work from home or keep regular hours while managing their migraine. Noise and light levels in the workplace can be reduced when possible and individuals with migraine should be permitted to take regular breaks during the day to manage their condition.

Other types of employer accommodations include providing a designated quiet area for individuals to be able to rest and relax when needed to manage their migraine. Additionally, if employees are required to travel for work, provisions can be made to bring medications and other supplies, such as noise-cancelling headphones, to ease the impact of migraine on the road.

Medical accommodations should also be provided. For instance, when an employee with migraine experiences a severe episode or the need for emergency medical treatment, the employer should be willing to provide time off from work and/or flexible scheduling to accommodate the needs of the employee.

Finally, employers should provide emotional support and

resources to employees with migraine. It is important to ensure that employees feel supported and encouraged to manage their migraine. A supportive dialogue between the employer and employee should take place to discuss the individual's various needs, strategize solutions, and explore other ways to support the individual's health. Moreover, employees should be provided with helpful resources such as access to support groups, online education and resources, and mental health therapies.

Dealing with Stress at Work

For the millions of people living with this disorder, one of the primary concerns is finding ways to effectively manage migraine in the workplace. In today's fast-paced business environments, stress is a real issue that can trigger the symptoms of migraine in many individuals.

Therefore, understanding the stress-migraine link is crucial to managing it effectively at work. Oftentimes, stress can be a factor in migraine development and can exacerbate existing conditions. Common sources of stress in the workplace include intense deadlines, long working hours, and little to no time off. Even a pleasant surprise, such as an extra assignment, can trigger migraine symptoms in some individuals.

There are certain steps that can be taken by individuals to help manage migraine in the workplace. First, it is important to assess the level of stress at work. Are there any tasks that can be pushed back or delegated so that the workload can be reduced? If so, those tasks should be removed or delegated to another team member. For those tasks that can't be removed, it can be helpful to break them down into smaller tasks and prioritize them in order of importance.

It can also be helpful to incorporate stress-reduction techniques into the workday, such as yoga, meditation, and deep breathing. These activities can not only help to reduce stress, but can also help to improve cognitive function so that tasks can be completed faster and at a higher quality. Additionally, it can be helpful to take short breaks throughout the day, such as a 10-minute walk or a cup of herbal tea.

In some cases, it may be necessary to make small adjustments to the work environment in order to prevent or reduce migraine symptoms. This can include increasing lighting and ventilation, keeping the temperature at a comfortable level, and allowing for some control over the noise levels in the office.

Finally, it is crucial to be good to oneself. Recognize stress-inducing activities and be kind to yourself by taking time to relax and unwind. Take mini vacations when possible, or look for ways to engage in activities that can improve overall health and wellbeing. All of these are important steps in managing migraine in the workplace.

CHAPTER TEN

Living with Migraine

Living with migraine can be challenging, and finding support is essential. Supportive communities can offer the needed reassurance and advice that can help patients cope with the physical and psychological impact of the chronic illness. There are a variety of different ways that patients with migraine can find support including self-help groups, online support networks, and in-person support groups.

Self-Help Groups

Self-help groups are a form of mutual support in which people affected and living with migraine come together to discuss their experiences and provide each other with support. One of the advantages of a self-help group is that members are able to hear from others who have gone through the same experiences. Group members also benefit from the support and advice of health professionals working with the group.

Online Support Networks

The internet has opened up new opportunities for people with migraine to find support. Online support networks provide an opportunity for patients, family members, and friends to connect, share experiences, and offer support. These networks may be based on specific support groups, websites, chatrooms, or forums. It is important to note that there are also many support networks available for specific types of migraine, such as chronic migraine, migraine with aura, and episodic migraine.

In-Person Support Groups

In-person support groups are a great way for patients with migraine to connect with others in person. Support groups may be hosted by local healthcare organizations, patient advocacy organizations, medical centers, or other health-related organizations. In-person support groups can provide an opportunity for people with migraine to connect with those dealing with similar experiences, gain advice from healthcare professionals, and even receive emotional support from fellow group members.

CONCLUSION

Everyone's experience is different and some people's migraines may not be as severe as others. For those living with more severe and frequent migraines, it is important to find medical guidance and appropriate care. Regardless of the severity, lifestyle changes, triggers management, natural remedies, and preventative medications can all play a part in helping to successfully manage these headaches.

Living with migraines can be a challenge, but many people are able to find relief with the right strategies and treatments tailored to their individual situation. The good news is, by focusing on triggers, preventative treatments, and lifestyle changes, migraine relief can be found.

The journey to finding migraine relief can be a long and complex one, but it is possible. For those with severe migraines, the journey may sometimes involve medical trials and errors. However, it is worth persisting and speaking to your doctor to find the best course of action for you.

As frustrating as it may be, it's important to remember that migraine relief may take some time. It may take several months to try different treatments and determine which one works best for you. However, with patience and dedication, it can be done. Ultimately, the goal is to minimize the frequency and intensity of your migraine headaches, and to maximize the quality of your life.

In conclusion, despite the challenges that migraines may have on our lives, it is possible to live with and manage them in a way that allows us to live a quality lifestyle. In order to do so, it is important to keep an open dialogue with your doctor and listen to their advice on treatments and lifestyle changes that will work best for you.

The journey to migraine relief can seem daunting at first, but it is possible and many have found relief from their migraine headaches. If you focus on learning more about your migraine triggers, taking preventative treatments, and making lifestyle changes, you can start on your own journey to finding migraine relief.